T'Was a Time Before Covid...???

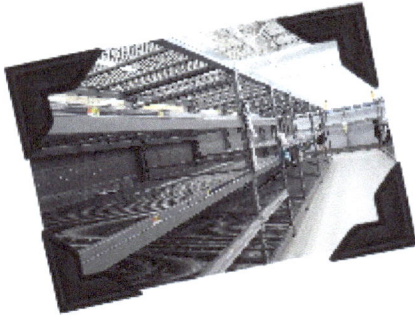

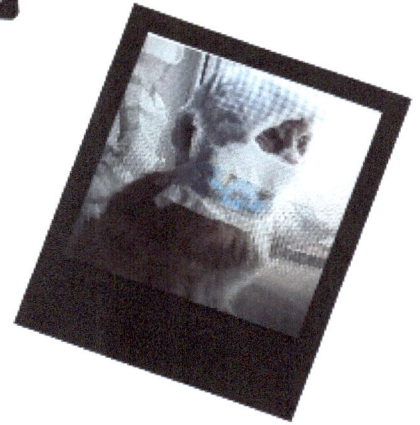

'Twas the year 2020, when all across
the world,
A pandemic of Covid intensely swirled.

The economy shut down, schools were closed,
People lost jobs, unemployment rates rose.

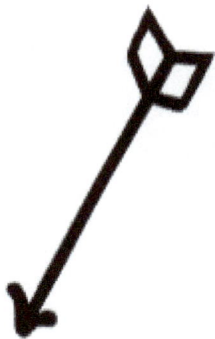

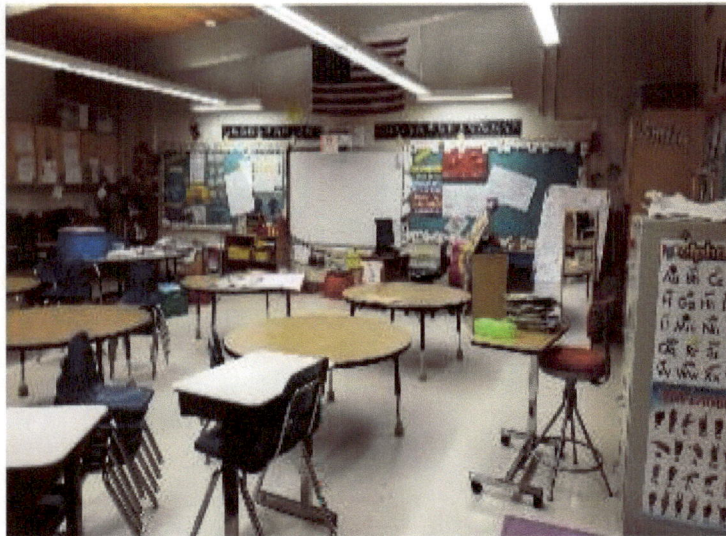

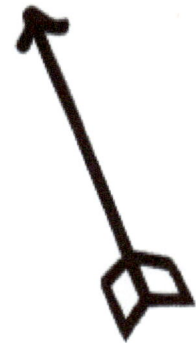

Day 1 of Homeschooling: Need the paperwork to get this kid transferred to another class.

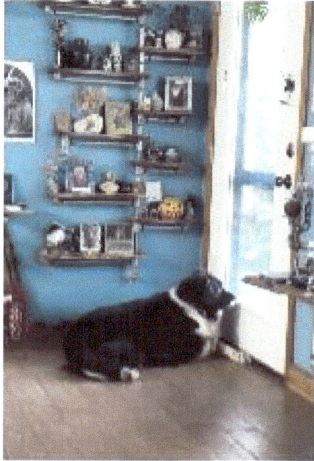

The government
ordered, we must
shelter in,
social distancing
and remote learning
were about to begin.

And Mother in her
mask, and I in my
N95,
Another new normal,
corona would contrive.

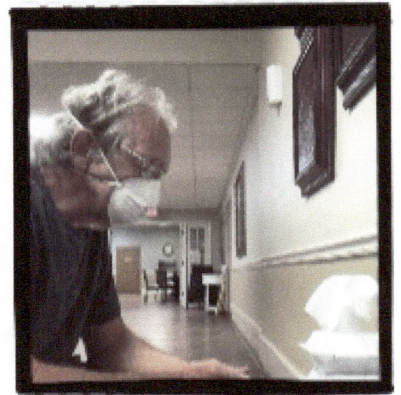

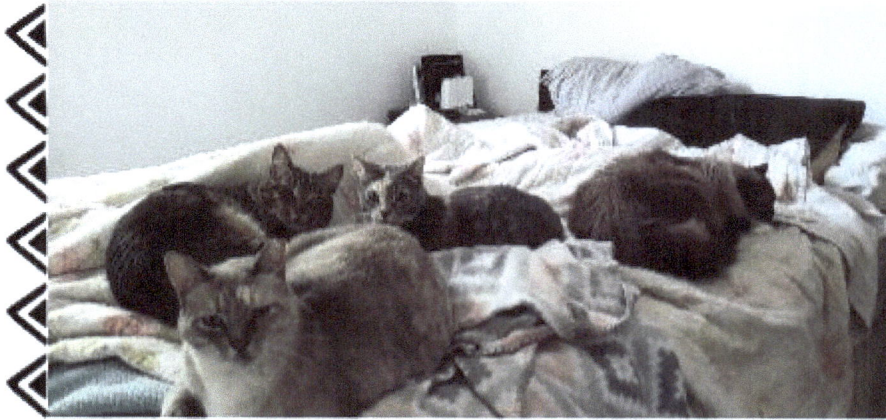

In case you lost track, today is April 16th

The President, Governors and Mayors all clattered,
We are in this together, flattening the curve is what mattered.

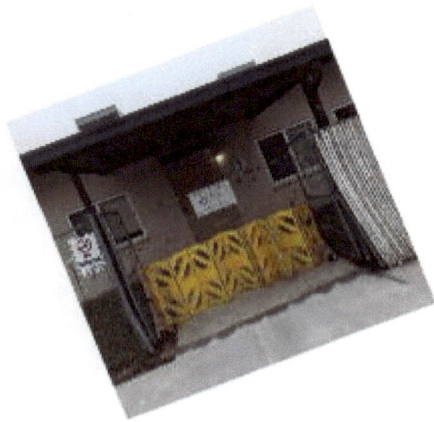

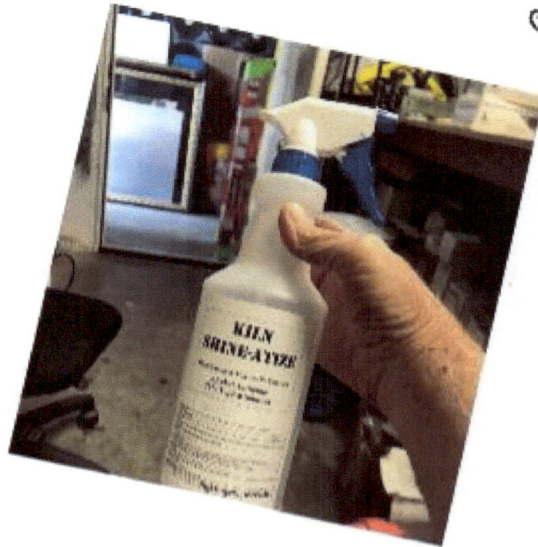

Fevers and coughing, the numbers soared in a flash,
Gathering sanitizer and gloves, washing hands till they rash.

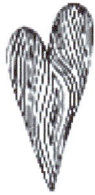

Hospitals and nursing homes
are in desperate need,
But they lack not for
heroes, fulfilling their
creed.

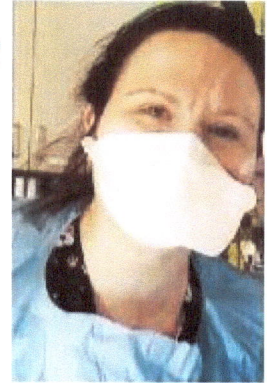

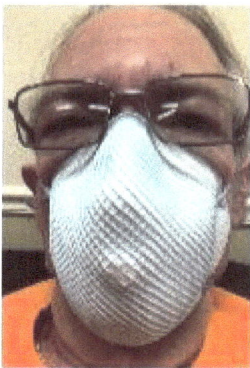

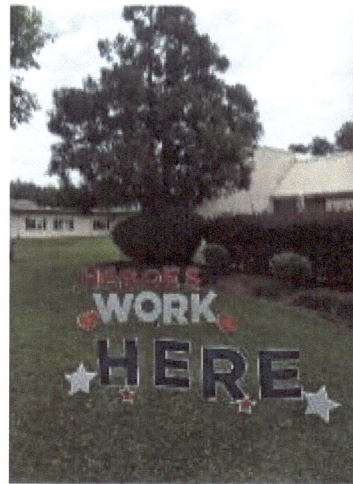

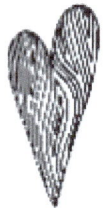

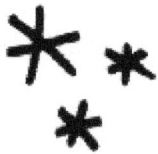

When what do the
rolling news updates
reveal,
But a slow in the
curve, announced with
great zeal.

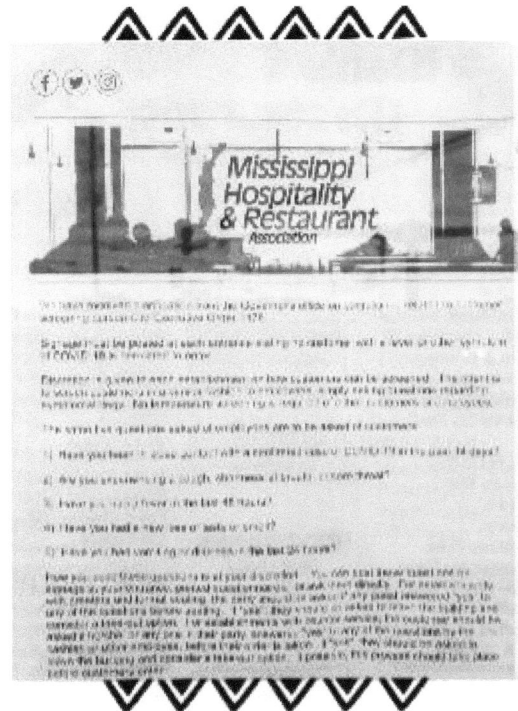

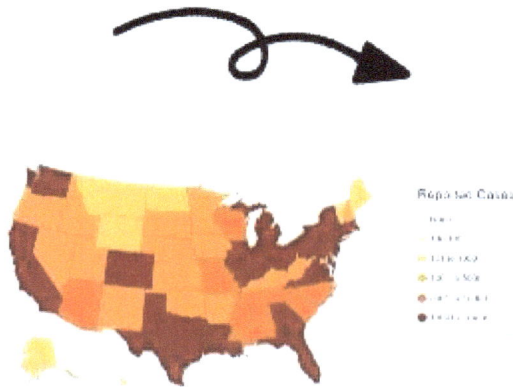

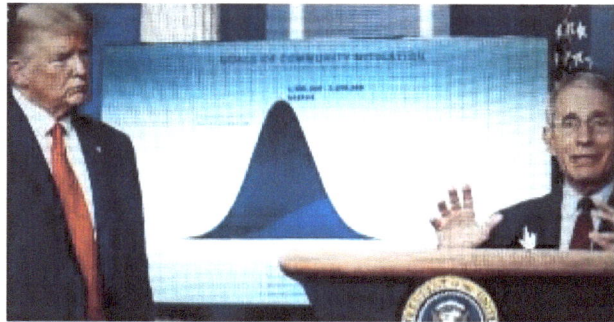

With reopen plans varying from
cities to states,
CDC guidelines, Trump's phases
determine the dates.

Cantrell cancels Jazz Fest, Essence and Voodoo.

Weddings, funerals and graduations scrapped too!

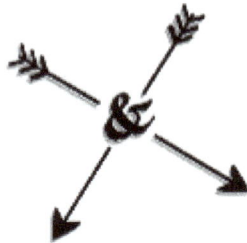

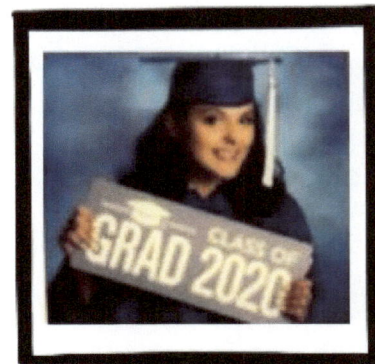

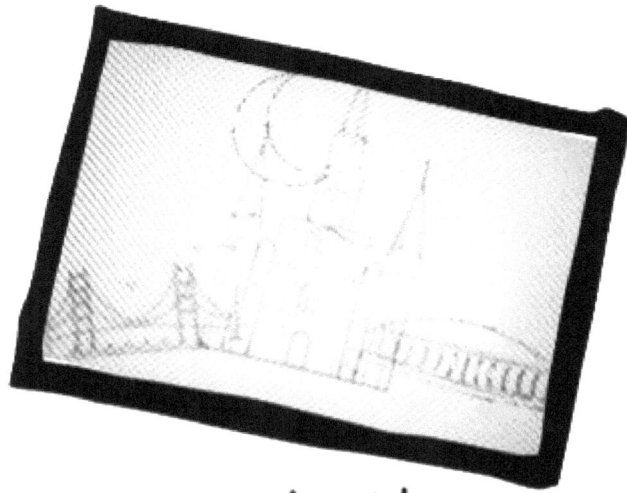

Restrictions are eased, the news
calls out names,
But our city's not ready, Mayor
Cantrell exclaims.

BANK STATEMENT

4/29/20   IRS TREAS $2,400.00

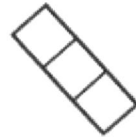

Unemployment checks, stimulus
money, vaccines and masks,
Could Mardi Gras be next, cut from
Orleans' future tasks?

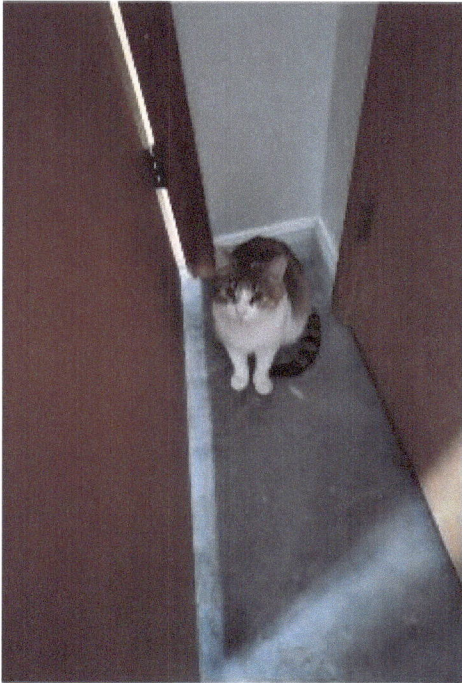

Testing and tracking, managing and care,
Closures and protesters, who decides what's fair?

Opinions, conspiracy
theories and
speculations all fly,
How long can this
last without our
economy's demise?

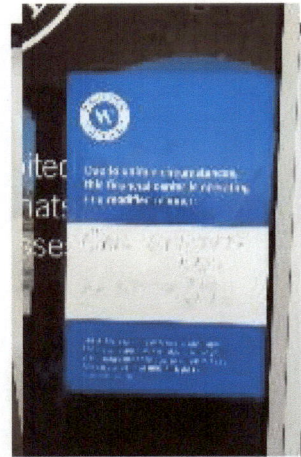

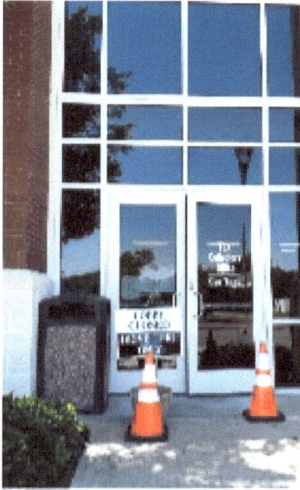

Headlines boast of unemployment benefits, Renters can't pay and landlords can't evict.

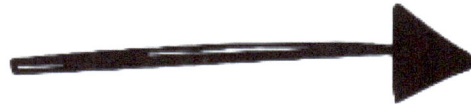

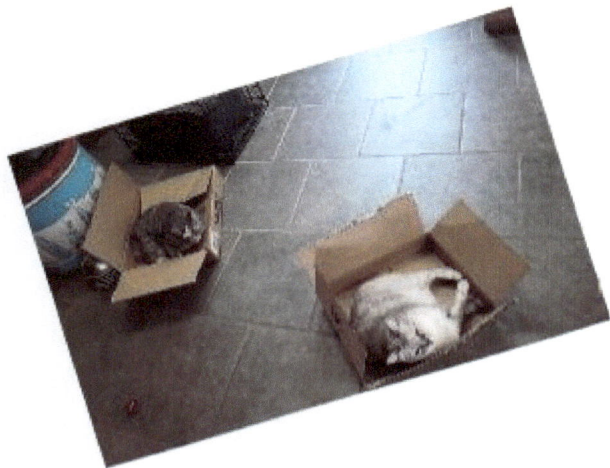

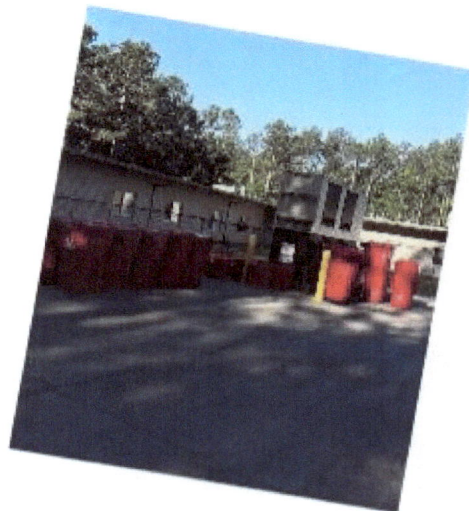

Safety precautions, Zoom meetings
and recommendations,
No church gatherings, no childcare,
but we have new legislation.

What makes a worker essential, and which ones are not, Aren't all Americans important in this Covid plot?

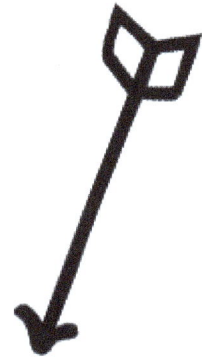

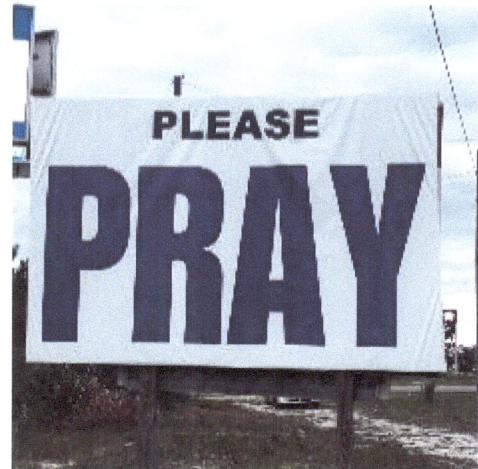

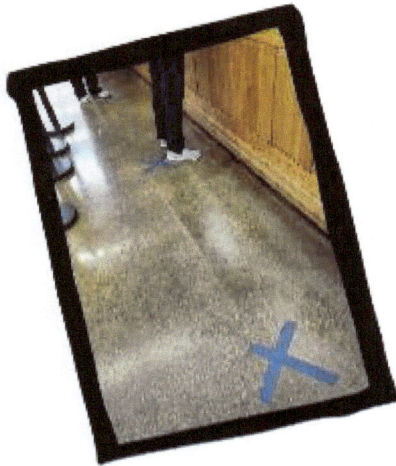

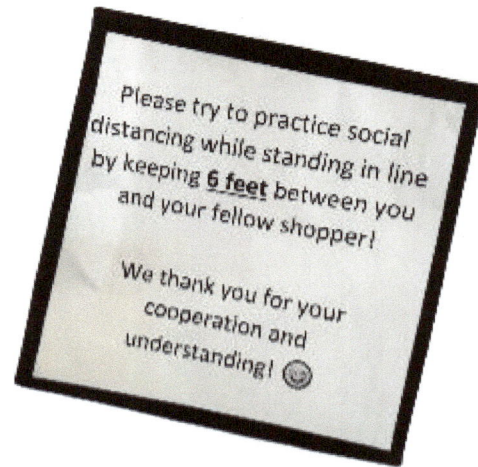

Please try to practice social distancing while standing in line by keeping **6 feet** between you and your fellow shopper!

We thank you for your cooperation and understanding! ☺

Shaking hands as a greeting or a goodbye as you depart,
No longer possible if we must stay six feet apart.

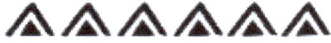

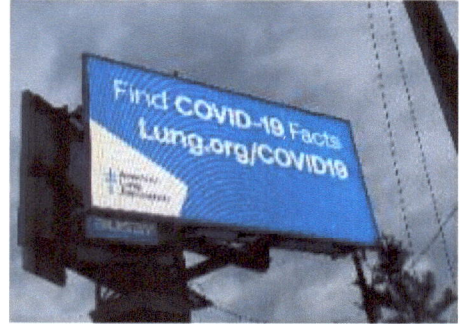

Why is Covid here,
when will it go,
If anyone holds the
truth, doesn't mean
we'll ever know.

April 45, 2020

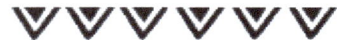

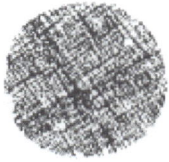

Lives need to flourish,
we can't live in fear,
Will the Covid, like
flu, come back every
year?

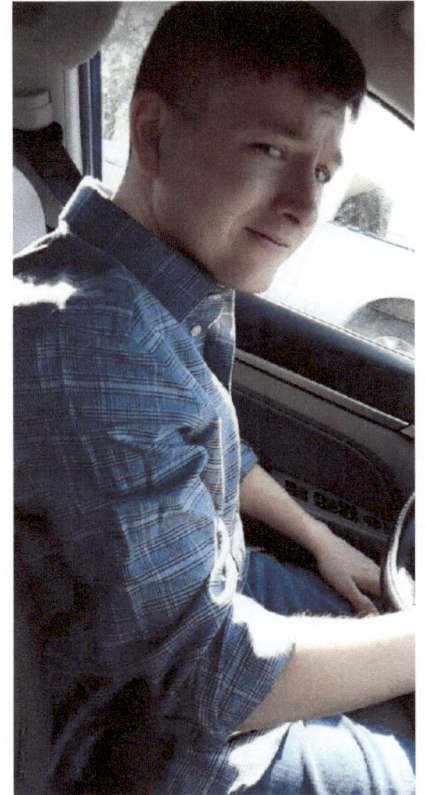

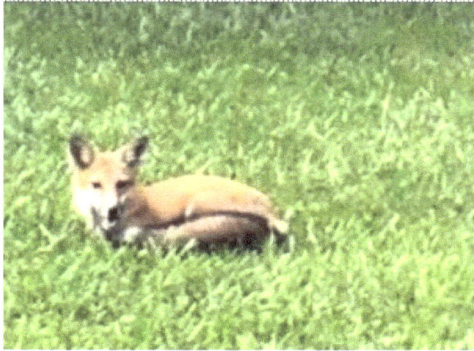

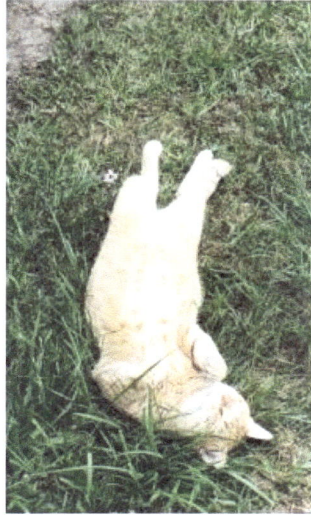

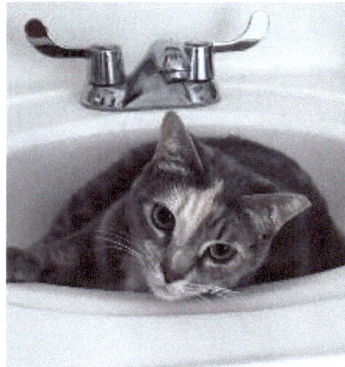

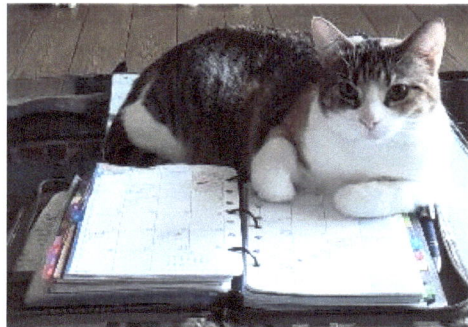

Laugh a Little
Try to Destress
Wash Your Hands
and
Do Your Best!

Pandemic Pondering

*#1 Throw Back Song - Don't Stand So Close To Me

* Dating Websites: Match, e harmony and now...
Contract Tracing

*Mask are the new fashion statement

*Restaurant Reservations - No worries
curbside pick-up and you get the best seat in YOUR
house

*2025 Attorneys offering class action lawsuits due
to health disorders from an over exposure of hand
sanitizer

_____

www.ingramcontent.com/pod-product-compliance
Lightning Source LLC
Chambersburg PA
CBHW052049190326
41521CB00002BA/161